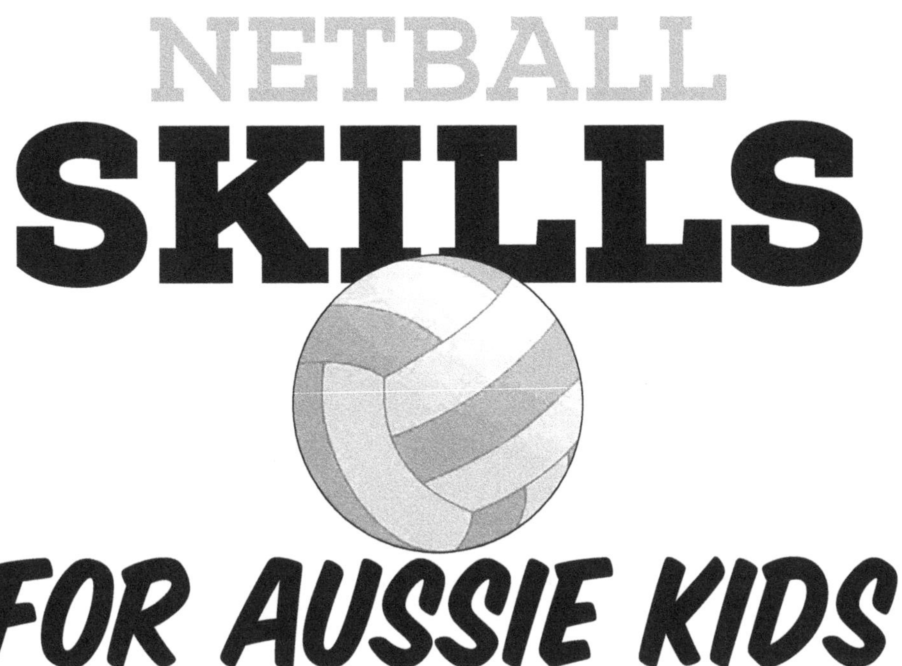

GARRY POWELL

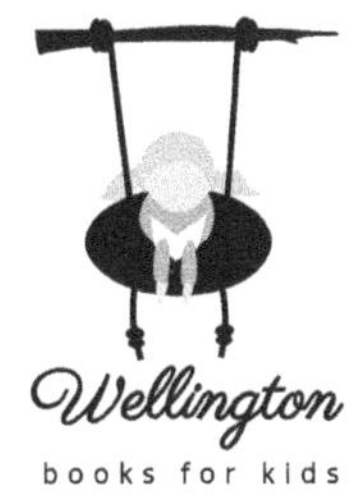

Netball Skills for Aussie Kids

ISBN: 978-1-922872-18-0 (paperback)
ISBN: 978-1-922872-19-7 (digital online)

Wellington (Aust.) Pty Ltd
ABN 30 062 365 413
433 Wellington Street
Clifton Hill
VIC 3068

CONTENTS

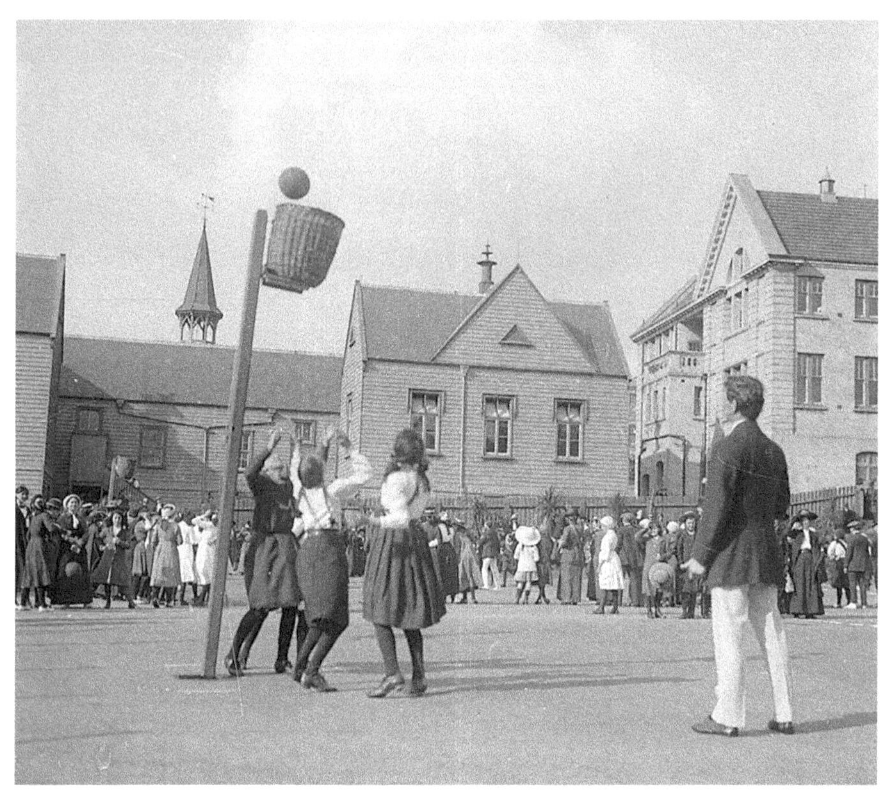

1910 Netball game in New Zealand

HISTORY OF THE GAME

The game of netball is based on basketball. Basketball was developed by Canadian Dr James Naismith in 1891 in Massachusetts, USA. By 1899 there were three sets of rules for basketball in the USA, including Spalding's 'Rules for Women'.

The first official set of rules for women's basketball were drawn up in 1901. These included the three-court system and the scoring of points instead of goals (depending on from where the shot was taken). This game soon spread to England and Jamaica.

Women's basketball was brought to Australia from England by women teachers in the early 1900s. At that time, there weren't many sports for girls played at schools, as it was thought that highly competitive sport for girls was 'not proper'. Women's basketball was thought to be more of an exercise rather than a sport. It became the main game for girls in schools throughout England and Australia.

In 1927 the All Australian Women's Basketball Association was formed, and the game spread due to the powerful women in charge of the sport.

In countries of the old British Commonwealth, netball is still the main winter sport for girls.

The name of the game was changed from women's basketball to netball in 1970.

The world championship in netball titled the World Cup was started in 1963 and is held every four years. Australia and New Zealand have dominated this competition in recent times.

Netball was first played in the Commonwealth Games in 1998.

THE COURT

Goal ring
Goal circle
Goal third
Centre third
Centre circle
Goal third
Sideline
4.9 m
30.5 m
10.2 m

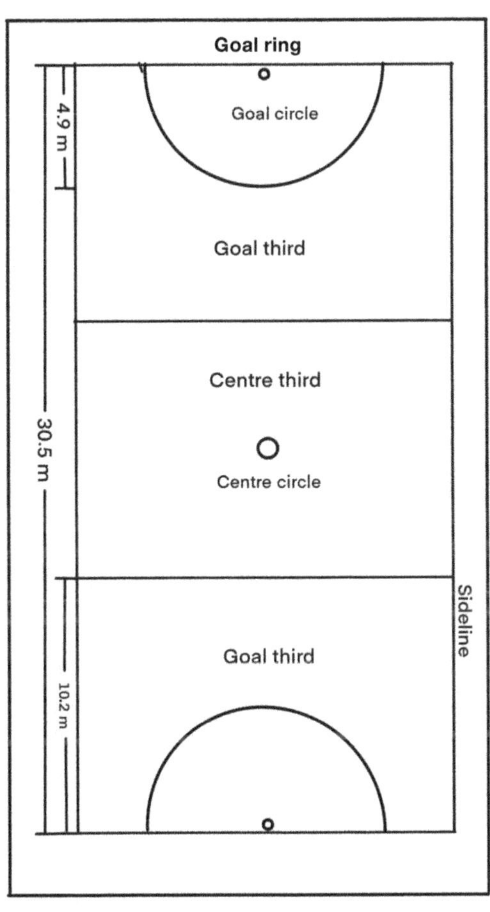

BASIC SKILLS

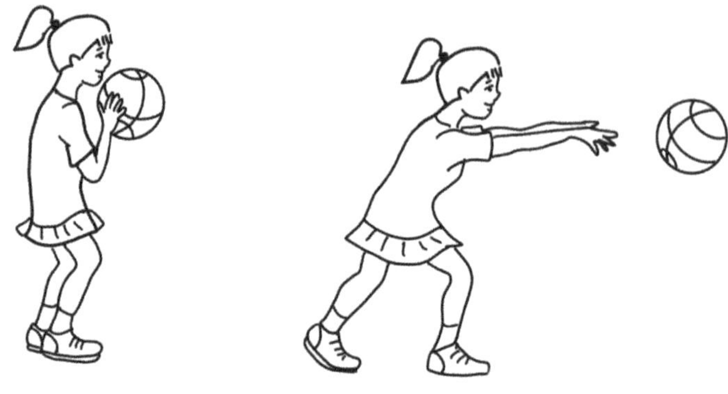

Throw

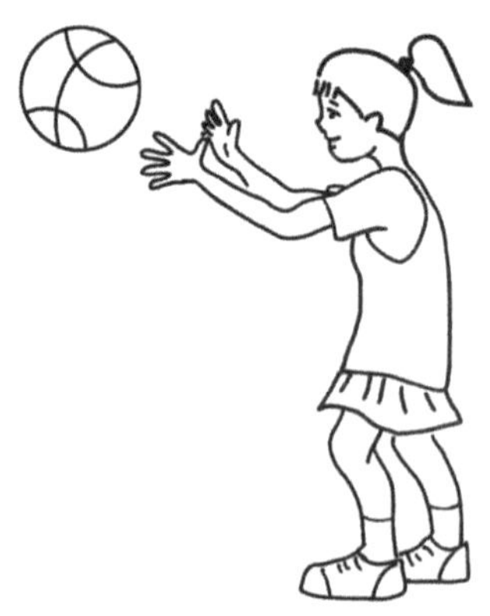

Catch

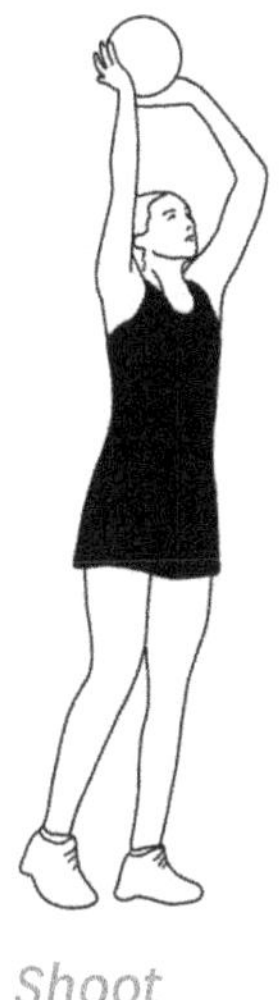

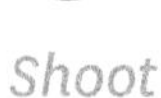

Shoot

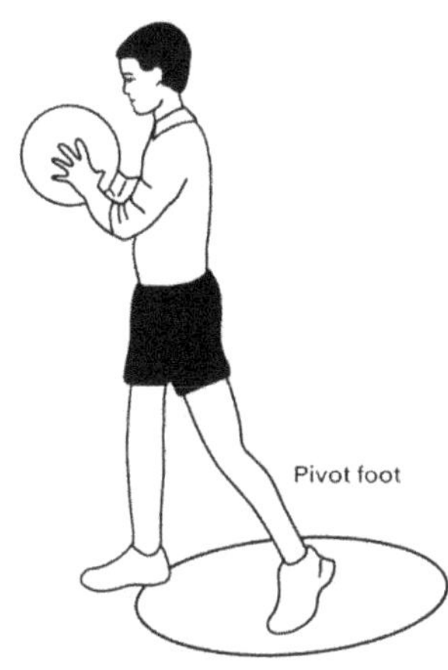

Pivot

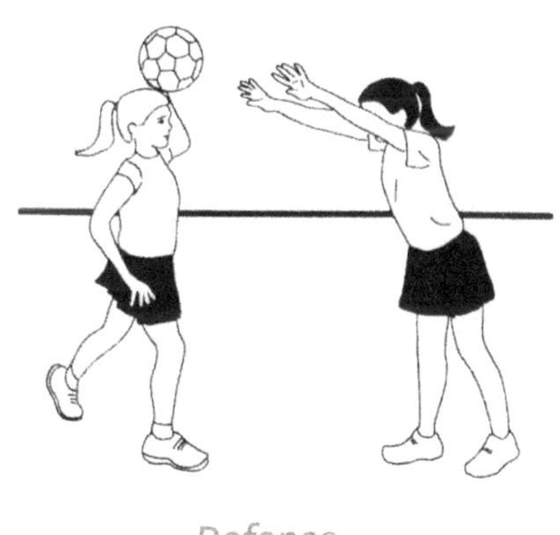

Defence

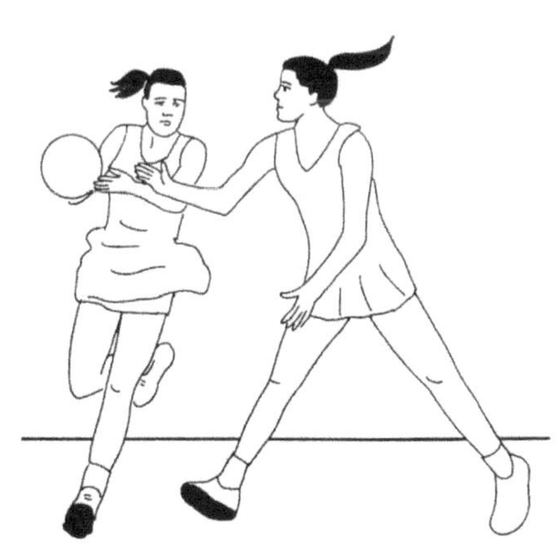

Attack

PASSING

Netball is basically a throwing and catching game. Throws to teammates are called passes.

Chest pass

This is a two-handed throw, which is the easiest pass.

→ Hold the ball in front of your chest. Look at your target.

→ Hands are held at the back of the ball with fingers spread evenly and thumbs pointing towards each other. Your hands are in contact with the lower half of the ball – the same position as if catching it.

→ Bring the ball close to your chest by bending your elbows.

→ Step forward and at the same time push the ball at the target with your arms straightening. The ball is released by a final flick of your fingers.

→ Your hands follow through towards the target.

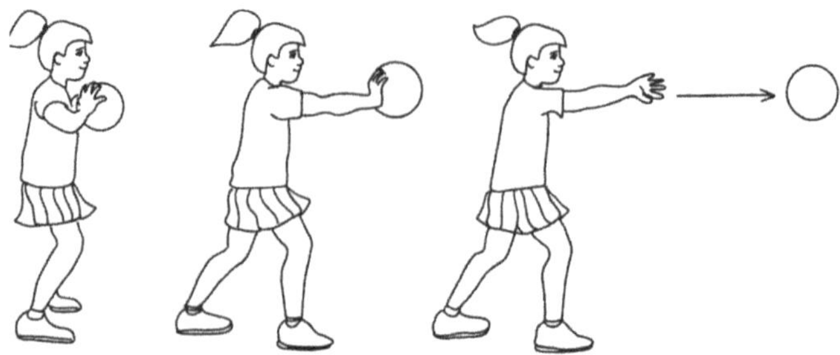

Chest pass

Shoulder pass

This is a one-handed throw used for longer passes.

- → At first the ball is held with both hands.
- → With the throwing hand the ball is taken back to near your ear.
- → Look at your target.
- → Step forwards on the foot opposite the throwing side (if throwing right-handed, step with the left foot).
- → At the same time, push the ball towards the target using your arm, shoulder and fingers.
- → Your throwing hand follows through towards the target.

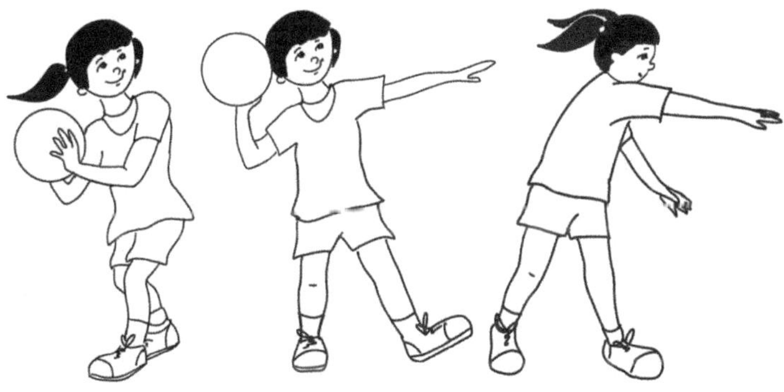

Shoulder pass

Overhead pass

This isn't used as much as the chest or shoulder passes, as it is not as accurate as a chest pass and cannot travel as far as a shoulder pass. It is mostly used when an opponent is nearby.

→ With elbows bent to about your ear level, hold the ball above your head.

→ Place your feet about shoulder width apart.

→ Look at your target.

→ Aim at high on your teammate's chest to make it easy to catch.

→ Just before you step forward, lower the ball so that it is just behind the top of your head.

→ Take a step towards your target and swing your arms forward from your shoulders.

→ Release the ball with a flick of your wrists.

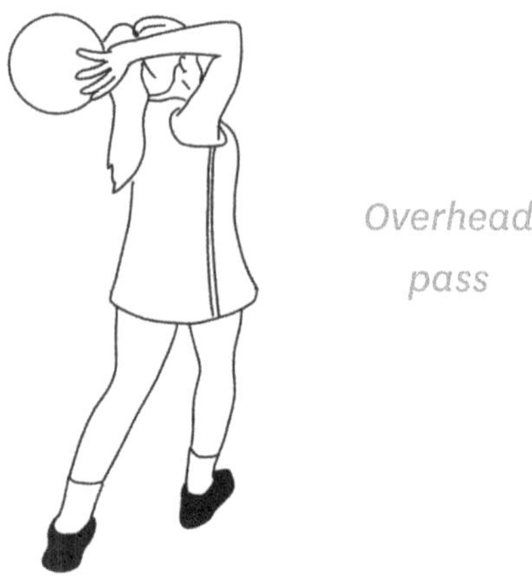

Overhead pass

Lob pass

This is a ball thrown in a high arc to travel over an opponent.

- → This pass is usually made using one hand, but can also be done with two hands.
- → Hold the ball above and behind your head.
- → Face your target.
- → Step forward towards the target.
- → At the same time, stretch your throwing arm up and forward towards the target.
- → The ball leaves your hand with a flick of your wrist and fingers.
- → Your throwing arm follows through high along the path of the ball.

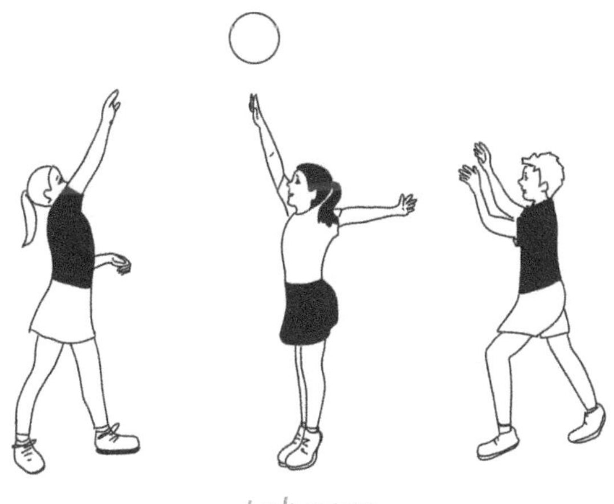

Lob pass

Bounce pass

This is a pass aimed to go under a close opponent's arm, and is only used for short passes.

- → At first the ball is held in both hands.
- → The passer chooses a spot on the ground at which to aim the ball – about two-thirds of the way to the teammate.
- → Look at this target spot.
- → At about hip level, the ball is shifted to the throwing hand.
- → Bend your knees, take a step forward and push the ball to the ground.
- → Your hand follows the line of the ball.
- → The ball should travel under the opponent's arm to land on the ground on the chosen spot, and then bounce up for your teammate to catch.

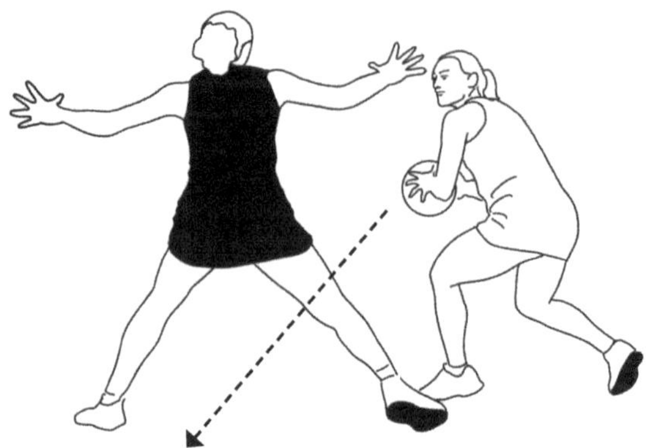

Bounce pass

CATCHING

Standing catch

- → Watch the ball and work out when it will reach you.
- → Move your body to be in line and in front of the ball's flight path.
- → Stretch both arms out in front, fingers spread, thumbs pointing towards each other.
- → Watch the ball all the way into the fingers.
- → To complete the catch, 'give' with the arms and bring the ball closer to your chest and into the 'hold' position.
- → Be ready to pass the ball immediately.

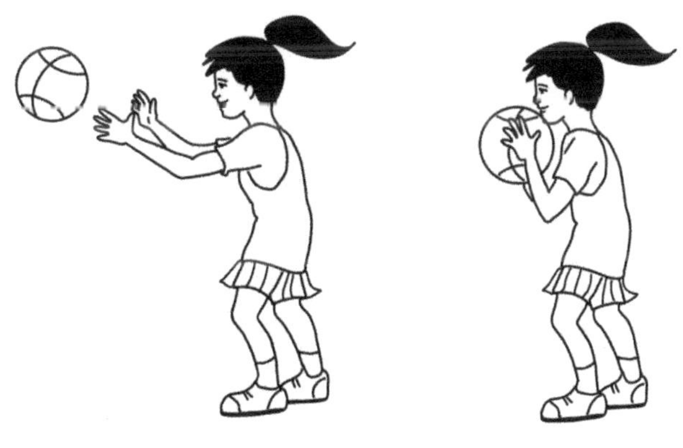

Standing catch

High catch

→ Watch the ball.

→ Move your body to be in line with the ball's flight path.

→ Stretch both arms above your head, fingers spread with thumbs pointing towards each other.

→ Keep extending your arms to reach the ball until they are almost straight.

→ Arms 'give' by bending at the elbows when the ball reaches you, and hands and fingers grip the ball.

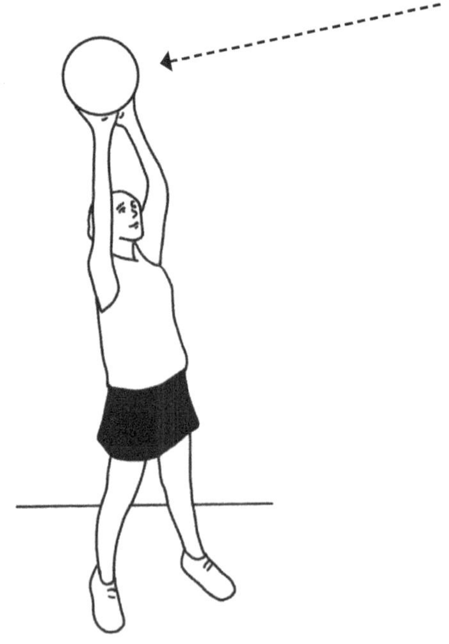

High catch

Jump catch

A jump catch is when a player catches the ball when in the air, having anticipated the path of the ball.

- → Watch the ball to anticipate where and when to jump to receive the ball.
- → Choose whether to lead with a jump off one or two feet.
- → Jump in the air towards that spot to receive the ball with arms and hands extended.
- → Keep arms slightly bent to catch the ball.
- → Land on both feet with knees bent to absorb body weight.

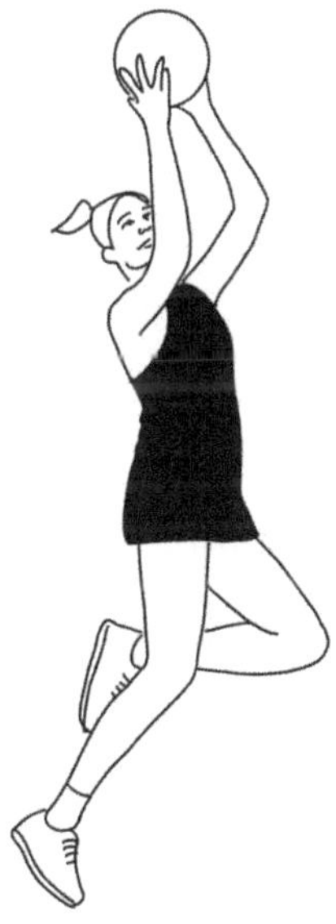

Jump catch

Running catch

Many catches have to be made 'on the run', as teammates often pass the ball to a space into which you can move ahead of your opponent.

→ Watch the ball.

→ Run towards the spot where you anticipate you will be able to catch it.

→ As the ball comes closer, stretch your arms in a relaxed manner towards it.

→ Grasp the ball with fingers and hands.

→ As contact is made with the ball, 'give' with your arms to accept the force of the ball.

→ If a jump is needed to reach the ball, bend your knees when landing to absorb your body's weight.

→ If heading to the right, the catcher tries to land on the right foot; and if running to the left, the left foot. This is because the landing foot cannot be lifted until the ball is passed again.

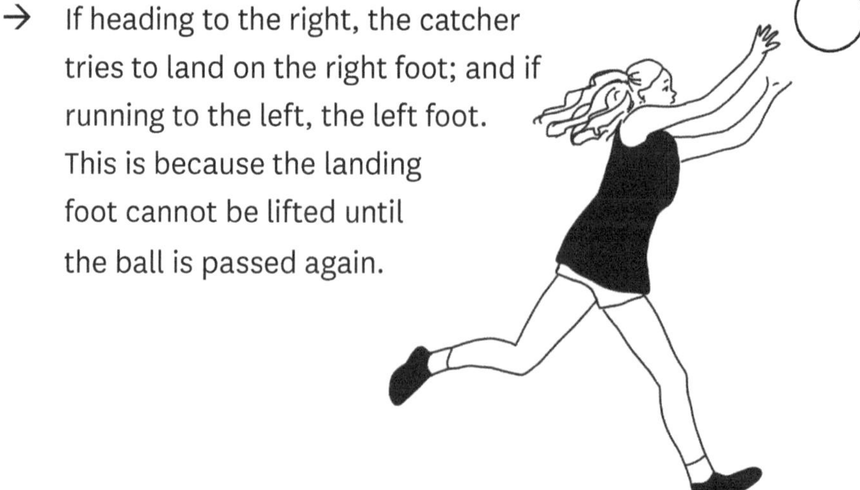

Running catch

SHOOTING

Shooting for goal is an important skill for all to have. There are only two goal shooting positions in a team, but any team member may be elected to play in these positions.

→ Stand tall and face the goal.

→ Set feet a comfortable distance apart.

→ Hold the ball overhead using both hands. The ball should be on the fingers and top half of the palm of the shooting hand. The non-shooting hand steadies the ball.

→ Take aim at the goal ring, and slightly bend at the knees and elbows in readiness.

→ Push up by straightening both legs and keeping the back straight as you shoot.

→ Shoot by taking non-shooting hand off the ball and the shooting arm pushing the ball with the wrist and fingers flicking the ball towards its target.

→ Follow through with shooting arm and fingers towards the ring, creating a loop shot with the ball.

→ Move quickly towards the goal after the shot in case of a rebound.

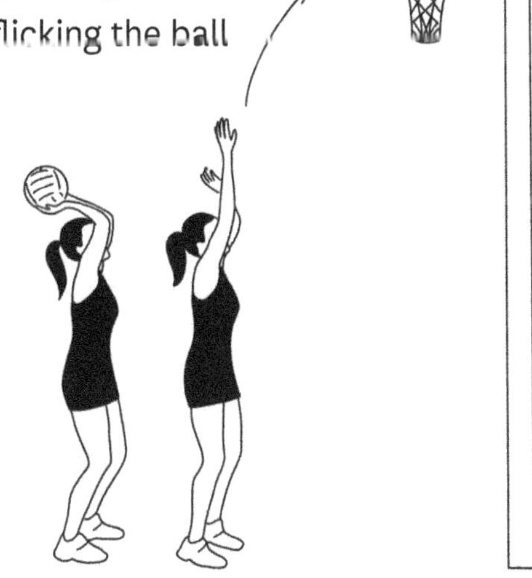

Standing shot at goal

PIVOT

In the game of netball, a player cannot take more than one step after getting possession of the ball. So balance and footwork are important skills.

A pivot is to swivel on one foot to change direction and take one step with the other foot. The pivot foot does not come off the ground.

The purpose of a pivot is to turn away from an opponent or to find and look at a teammate to whom you can pass the ball.

→ Hold the ball in front of your chest, whether it be after a standing catch or landing after a jump catch.

→ Keeping your pivot foot on the ground, take a step in another direction so you are facing in a different direction.

→ As long as your pivot foot doesn't lift, you can take multiple sidesteps with your free foot.

→ Your pivot foot can swivel, as long as it does not leave the ground.

→ All of this has to take place within the three seconds allowed before you must dispose of the ball.

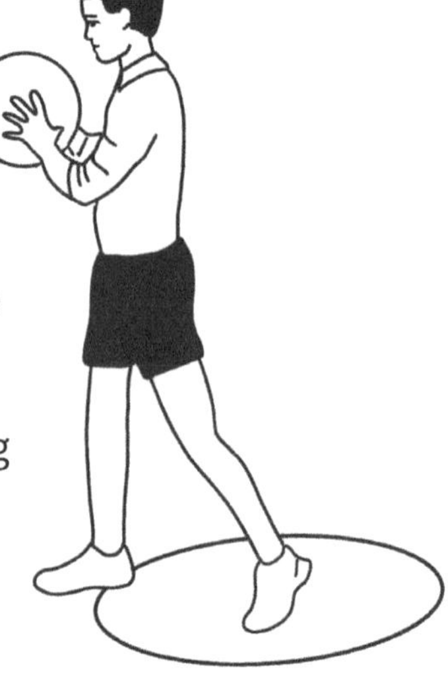

Pivoting on the left foot

ATTACK

When a team has possession of the ball, all members are attackers with the aim of getting the ball to a player who can shoot for goal.

Because in netball a player in possession of the ball can only take one step, most player movement comes before they get the ball.

Attacking in netball is about 'getting away' from your defending opponent, then 'getting into' into a free space into which a teammate can pass you the ball.

A good attacker changes their types of movement often so that the defender is 'kept guessing'.

Sprint

This is a sudden burst of speed from standing into a space ahead.

→ This action should be sudden and very fast.

→ It can be straight at your teammate who has the ball, or sideways into a space.

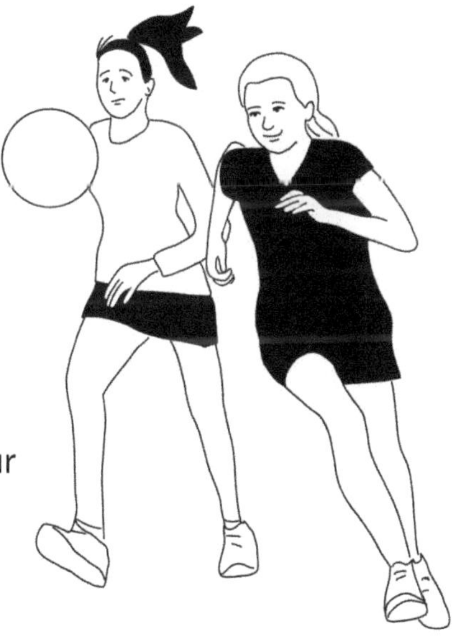

Sprint

Dummy

With the defender near you, lean in one direction and then push off hard with the weight on that foot and sprint in a different direction. The defender may have expected you to run in the direction you were leaning, and this gives you a start distance to get away.

→ Keep your head up, and when free in a space look at your teammate so you can see the ball come to you.

→ As soon as you are in a free space, get your hands in front of your chest ready to catch the incoming pass.

Dodge

This is a bigger movement than the dummy.

→ Change direction quickly when moving into a space to outmanoeuvre an opponent.

→ Take two, three or four steps in one direction and then quickly push off in the opposite direction with the foot on that side of the body.

→ Even if the attacker does not receive the ball, the space created with the movement can be used by teammates

DEFEND

All the defensive skills outlined here are for 'one-on-one' defence – that is, one defender on one attacker. When a team does not have possession of the ball, all players become defenders. Their aim could be to:

- → stop the attackers getting to shoot at goal
- → making the shot for goal difficult
- → gain possession of the ball from the attackers.

Marking

Marking is used to stop an attacking opponent getting the ball or getting into a free space to receive the ball. The marker moves in the same direction as the opponent to be able to intercept a pass. The defender cannot get closer than 0.9 metres to the attacking opponent as body contact is not allowed.

- → There are three ways to mark an attacking player.
- → Marking – is when a defender stands with back to the attacker, making the body as 'big' as possible by being on tiptoes and stretching arms out, without impeding the attacker. It is important to turn the head to watch both the attacker and the ball.
- → Close marking – is when a defender stands side-on, facing the attacking player. This allows sight of both

the attacker and ball at the same time. Being on the toes and balls of feet allows quick movement either way to anticipate a move or pass.

→ Double marking – is when two players mark a single opposing player to ensure that the player does not receive the ball. This happens often in the goal circle by marking one shooter. Care must be taken to avoid contact with the shooter.

Watch the eyes of the person with the ball to anticipate the direction of the throw.

To intercept the ball side-on, make sure it's always done with the arm furthest from the attacker to avoid contact.

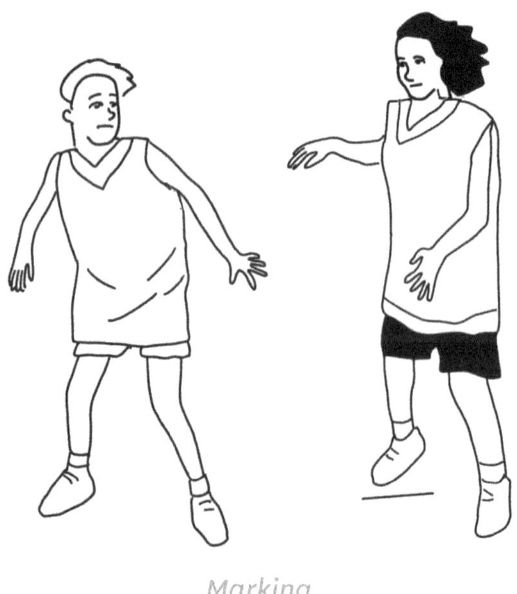

Marking

Intercept

To intercept means to interrupt a pass to or from an opponent. This could be knocking the ball down or away or gaining possession of an opponent's pass.

→ The key to success is to anticipate where the ball will be received and an opponent's direction of movement.

→ Quick movement in front of an opponent is needed to intercept by catching the pass, or to reach into the ball path from the side to knock the ball away from an attacker.

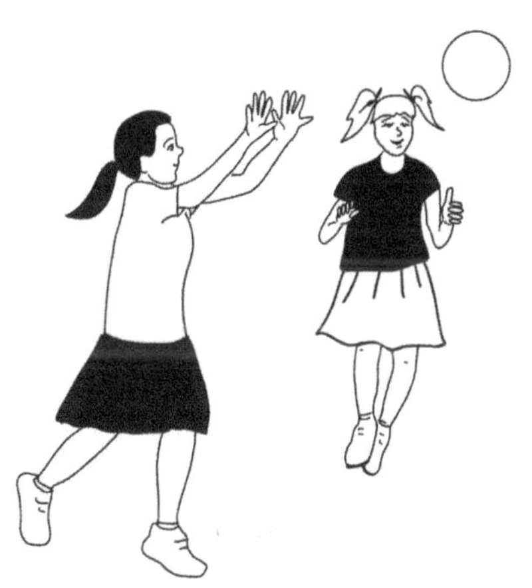

Intercept

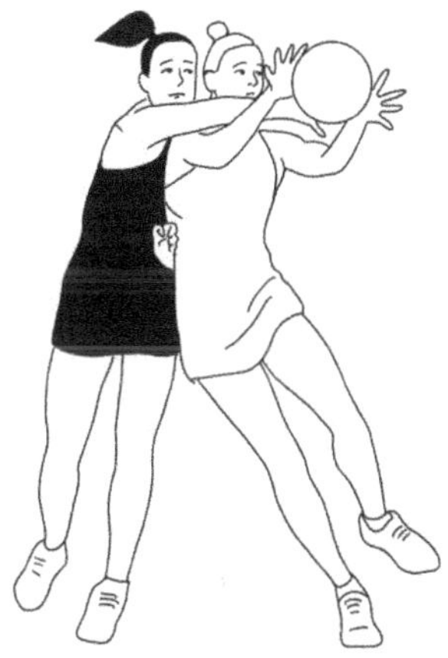

Reach into the ball path

Blocking

There are two types of blocking: making it difficult for an attacker to move into a space to receive a pass, and making it difficult for an attacker who has the ball to either pass or shoot at goal.

- → As for all netball plays, the defender must stay 0.9 metres away from their opponent and cannot deliberately touch them.
- → To block a player from an easy path to find space to receive the ball, the defender must be in front of the attacker.
- → The defender faces the attacker.
- → Each movement to get free by the attacker is matched by the defender, so that the attacker cannot get past.
- → If the ball is thrown, the defender tries to turn to block the ball with their hand.

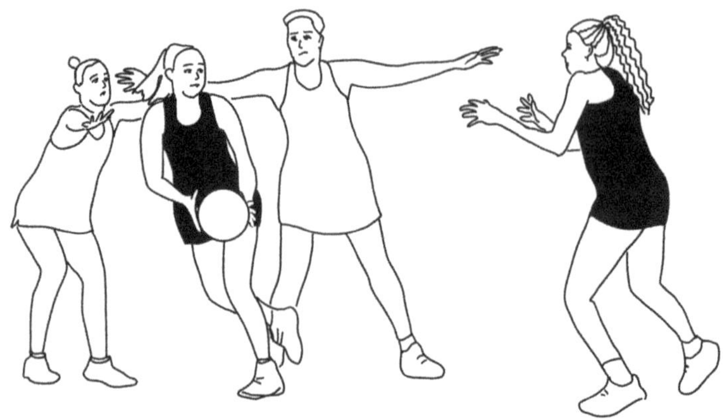

Blocking space

- To make a shot at goal more difficult: The defender stands as tall as possible.
- One arm reaches up to try to block the flight of the ball.
- You can jump up to try to touch the ball, as long as you stay 0.9 metres away from the attacker.

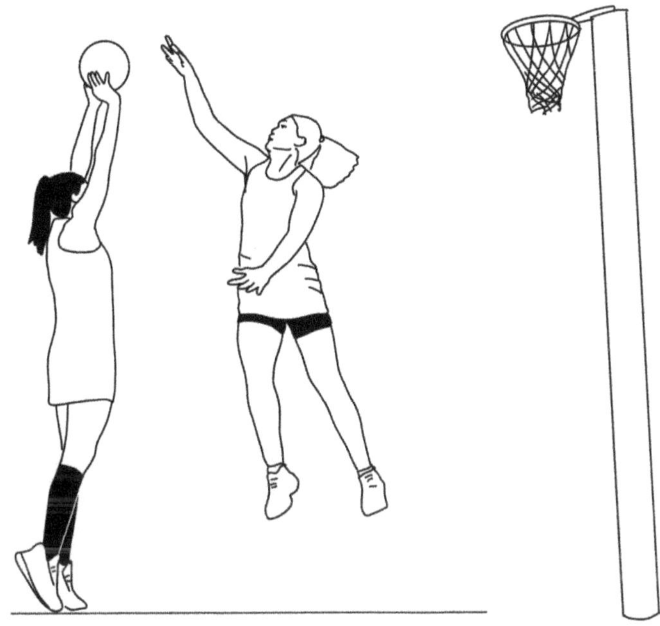

Blocking a shot at goal

HARDER SKILLS

In netball games for older children and adults, team attack and defence is used as well as individual skills. Some of the more difficult individual skills are demonstrated below.

PASSING

Side pass

The side pass is used to avoid a blocking opponent.

- → Hold the ball with both hands in front of your face.
- → Bring the ball back over one shoulder until the front of the ball is level with the back of your head.

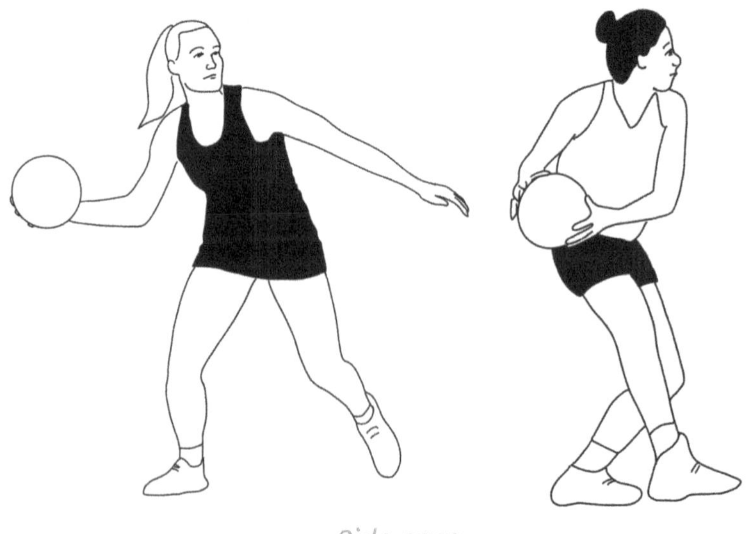

Side pass

- Lean to one side to avoid your opponent.
- Step forward as you release the ball.
- Throw the ball with power progressing from your shoulder – arms – both hands – throwing hand and wrist.

Jump pass

This is a shoulder pass while running that prevents incorrect footwork on landing.

- Look at the target.
- Leap into the air off one foot.
- Draw the ball back using the hand opposite the jump foot.
- With both feet off the ground, a strong shoulder pass is done.
- The landing can then be either on one or two feet, as you no longer have possession of the ball.

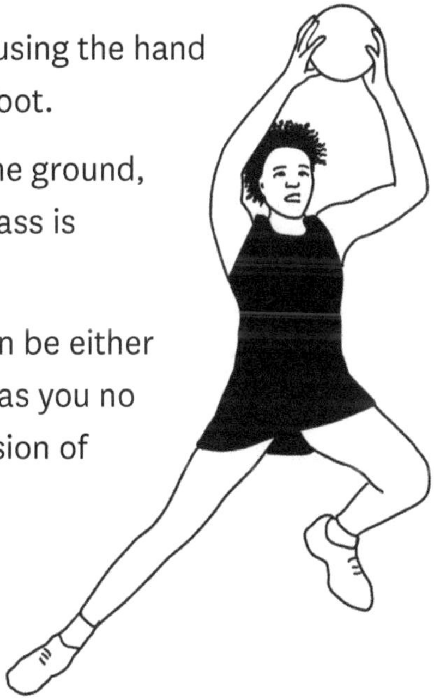

Jump pass

One-hand catch

When a two-handed catch is not possible for a high or side ball, the one-hand catch is taken with an extended arm and one hand.

- → Watch the ball to judge where and when the flight of the ball will be closest.
- → Extend the arm closest to the flight of the ball with hand ready to catch it.
- → For a high ball, timing the jump to reach the ball at its highest point is important.
- → Quickly pull the ball in towards the chest so that it can be held firmly with both hands.

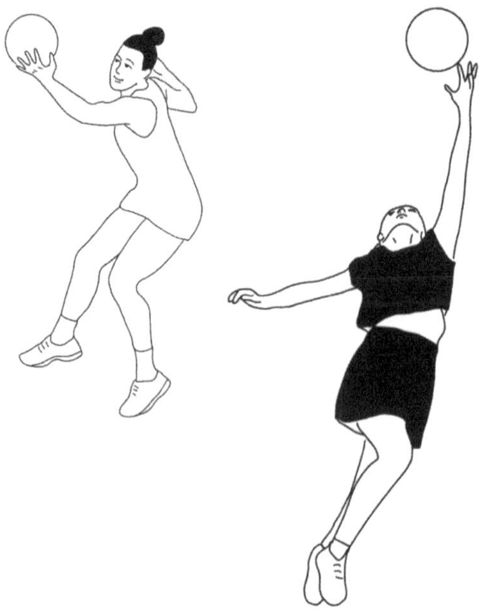

One-hand catch

SHOOTING

Jump shot

This is usually the end of receiving a pass while running.

→ On receiving the pass, the goal shooter may find that there are no defenders between themselves and the goal ring.

→ Using the footwork rule, a player may have one foot grounded, or jump into the air to be closer to the goal before shooting.

Step shot

→ If the shooter finds that the defender's hand blocks a direct path to the ring, the shooter can take one single step to the side or back before shooting. The aim of the step shot is to avoid defender interference on the ball and get a better sight and shooting line to the goal.

→ If the defender's hand blocks the shooting path after a moving or jumping catch into the goal circle, the shooter can use the non-landing foot, taking one step to the side or back, lifting the landing foot off the ground.

→ The shooter steadies, maintaining a balanced position on this leg and shoots for goal.

- → The defender cannot move closer than the 0.9 metres from the shooter's first grounded foot.

Rebound

A shot at goal may be unsuccessful and the ball can bounce off the goal ring.

- → Both defenders and attackers are allowed to attempt to catch this ball if it is still within the goal circle.
- → Defenders should be best placed to catch this rebounding ball as they can position themselves while the shot for goal is taken.

Jump – land – pivot

When a jump in the air is taken to catch the ball, the first foot to touch the ground is called the landing foot.

- → This foot can then be pivoted on to change the way you are facing.
- → This same landing foot can be lifted off the ground to start a step, but the ball must be released before the foot touches the ground again.

Toss-up

If two players catch, pick up or wrestle the ball at the same time, the umpire will stop play and a toss-up will take place.

- → The two players contesting the ball stand facing each other at least 0.9 metres apart.
- → The umpire throws the ball up between the two players, who jump to compete for the catch.
- → Normal play continues after one player gains control of the ball.

PRACTICE BY YOURSELF

THROWING/PASSING

All types of throws can be practised using these activities: chest, shoulder, overhead, lob and bounce. All throws can be with both right and left hands.

→ Throw against a wall.

→ Throw to hit a target on the wall.

→ Increase the distance of the throw.

→ Throw at a target from different angles.

→ Throw at a marked target to score points.

→ Throw over an obstacle to hit a target.

→ Throw from different body positions: standing front-on and side-on, kneeling and sitting.

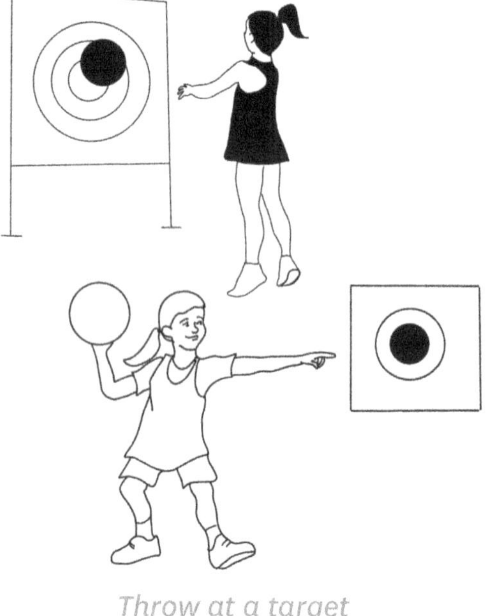

Throw at a target

CATCHING

All types of catches can be practised using these activities: chest, overhead, jump, one-hand.

→ Throw the ball into the air and catch it.
  - Throw into the air and clap once before the catch.
  - Throw and clap as many times as you can before the catch.
  - Catch the ball above your head.
  - Catch the ball with one hand.

→ Drop the ball and catch it.
  - Bounce the ball and catch it.
  - Bounce the ball so it goes high and catch it.
  - Bounce the ball high and catch it above your head.
  - Bounce the ball and catch with one hand.

→ Throw the ball against a wall and catch it.
  - Let the ball bounce before you catch it.
  - Catch it on the full.
  - Change the distance you stand away from the wall.
  - Throw the ball onto the ground so that it bounces against the wall and then catch the rebound.

→ Throw the ball into the air and catch it while you are walking.

- Walk forwards, sideways, backwards.
- Throw and catch while you are jogging – then running.
- Throw high, throw low, throw to the side, and run to catch.
- Repeat each exercise as many times as possible without dropping the ball.

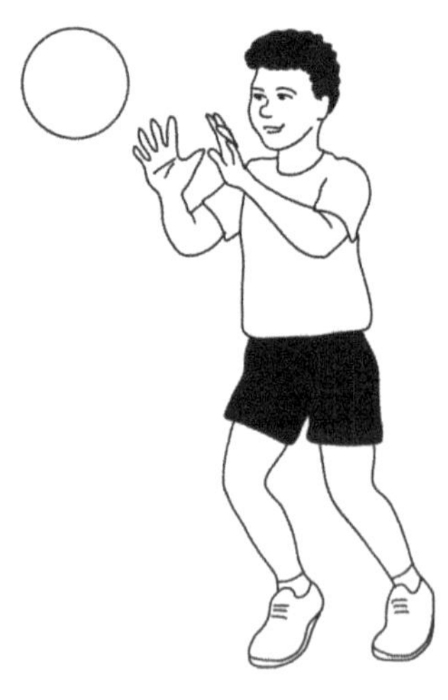

Catch

SHOOTING

Use a netball ring or a substitute, such as an old bike tyre, a bin or tin, a hoop, or even a mark on a wall.

- → Shoot from standing close to the goal ring.
- → Vary the distance from the goal.
- → Mark out a half goal circle and shoot from just inside the line.
- → Vary angles from the goal.
- → Shoot over a 'make believe' opponent.
- → Shoot with the preferred hand and then both hands.
- → Jump shot.
- → Step and shoot.

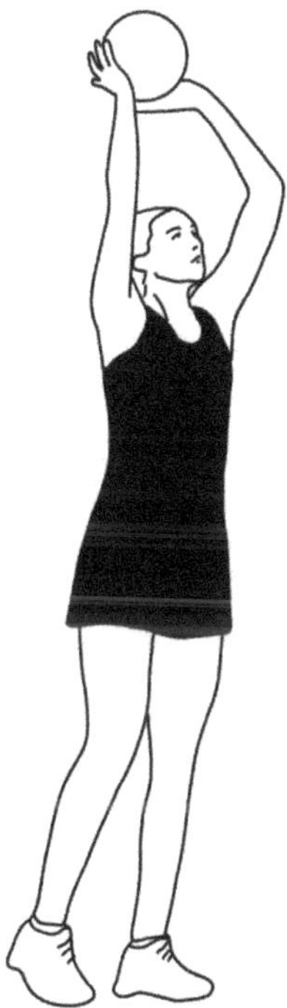

Two-hands shot

PIVOTING

→ Practise pivoting on both your left foot and your right foot, because both will be needed in a game situation.

→ Pivot near an imaginary opponent or use a marker as an opponent.

→ Pivot first without the ball, and then while carrying the ball.

→ Pivot from standing.

→ While holding the ball – jump into the air, then land and pivot.

→ Throw into the air, jump to catch the ball, land and pivot.

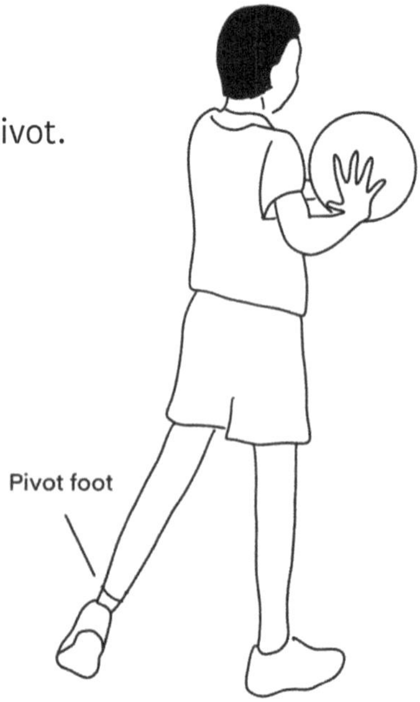

Pivot foot

Pivot away from a marker

ATTACK

Because in the game of netball you cannot take more than one step when in possession of the ball, the practices of attack and defend are basically agility exercises without the ball.

Sprint, dummy and dodge are the skills needed to 'get free' from an opponent.

- → Fast start – practise taking off fast from standing still.
- → Run fast for 3 metres from standing start, then for 5 metres, then for 10 metres.
- → Sidestep fast from standing.
- → Run backwards fast from standing.
- → Change direction – run fast in one direction for three steps, then change direction suddenly for another three steps.
- → Sprint away from and sidestep an imaginary opponent.
- → Rhythmic exercises: hopping, jumping, galloping, skipping, clapping, toe tapping, lunging, swinging arms or legs.
- → Standing long jump, high jump, hop-step-jump, as in athletics.
- → Naming and singing games with a skipping rope.

→ Use a marker as an opponent.

→ Dodge around an obstacle course.
Make different obstacle courses: in and out, around and back, zigzags, lanes, circles, tight turns.

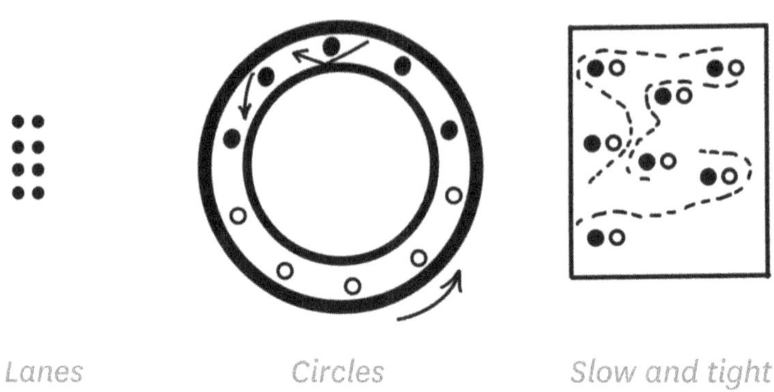

Lanes *Circles* *Slow and tight*

DEFEND

Mark, intercept and block are the three basic defence skills.

- → Mark and block an imaginary opponent.
- → Jump to touch an imaginary shot at goal.
- → Use a marker as an opponent.
- → Mark or follow an opponent by moving with the opponent in all directions.
- → Block an opponent with arms up, and/or back to an opponent, watching over their shoulder.

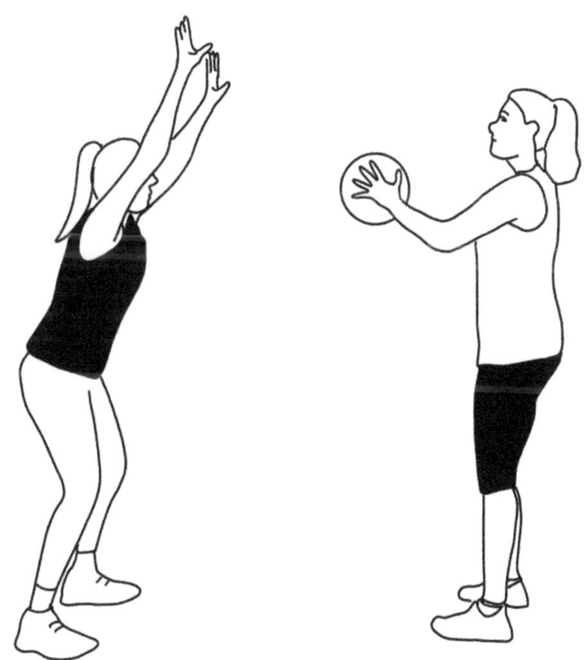

Blocking an imaginary shot at goal

- → Throw the ball in the air towards an opponent, and rush in to catch the ball before it gets to the opponent.
- → Throw the ball high towards the marker but knock it away before it gets there.

PRACTICE WITH A PARTNER

THROWING AND CATCHING

All types of passes and catches can be practised using these activities.

Throw: chest, shoulder, overhead, lob, bounce, side and jump.

Catch: chest, high, jump, running, one-hand.

→ Back to Back

- Standing back to back, the player with the ball (player A), twists around to their right to hold the ball out towards their partner.
- The partner (player B) twists to their left side to grasp the 'held out' ball.
- All four feet should remain 'stuck to the ground' and the ball should never be 'hands free'.
- Then player B twists to their right and player A to their left to receive the ball that has now travelled in a circle.

→ Do five circles in a row – then see if 10 circles can be made without a mistake.

→ Under and over – standing back to back, partners hand the ball to their partner back between their legs and it is returned back over their head.

- Throw to a partner from 1 metre apart.
- Vary the distance of the throws – 1, 5 and 10 metres.
- Throw to a partner while moving and the partner is stationary.
- Throw while both partners are moving – walking, jogging, running.
- All these passes should be practised at first using only one type of throw such as chest or bounce. The catch should be whichever is the most appropriate such as chest or one hand.
- Both the throw and the pass are nominated before the practice starts – this might make the catch more difficult, as it may not be the most appropriate depending on the ball's flight path.
- Examples can include a jump throw and a chest catch.

→ Ten Up – take turns to throw at a target – first to 10 hits is the winner.

→ Follow the Leader – take turns as leader – the leader chooses a type of throw and catch, and the partner has to follow.

This can be an individual throw and catch to themselves, or a type of throw and catch to each other.

- One partner shoots at goal and the other catches the rebound, whether it scores a goal or not. Change roles after a certain number of shots. This can be made a competition by counting the number of rebounds caught after 10 shots at goal.
- Progression Ball
  - Players start at an equal distance from a midline.

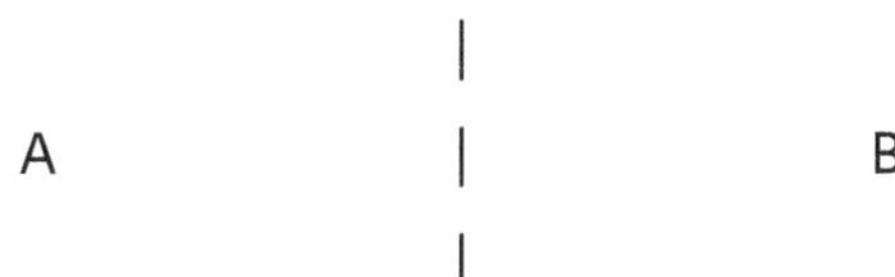

  - Partner A passes the ball to partner B. If this throw/pass allows partner B to touch the ball without moving, partner A takes a step backwards. Partner B then throws to partner A from their new starting distance. The winner is the partner furthest from the midline after an equal number of passes.
- Force Back
  - Partners start at an equal distance from a midline.

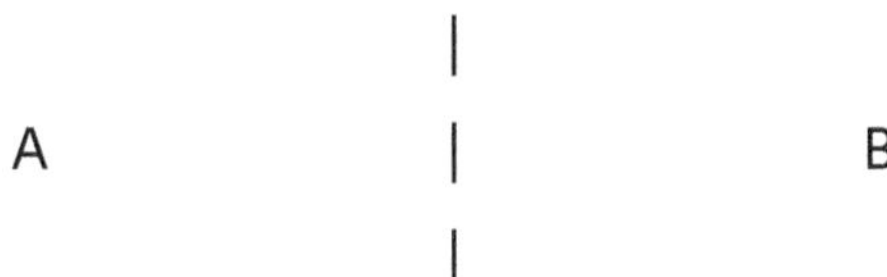

  - Partner A throws the ball towards partner B. This pass must have a landing point within 2 metres of B. If B catches the ball, they then throw the ball back towards A from exactly where it was caught. If the ball is not caught, B takes a step backwards along the throw line and A takes a step forward along the throw line. These positions now become their throw and catch points.

- The aim of this game is to force the partner back until they can catch the return throw on the opposite side of the midline from where they started.

Rebound Ball

→ Player A throws the ball at a wall and player B has to catch the return ball either 'on the full', or after one bounce.

→ The throw can be varied by: distance, height on the wall, or bounce pass.

→ After 10 successful catches, partners change roles.

Dodge the Blocker

→ Throw the ball to hit the target. This can be around or over the chair, depending on the thrower's starting position.

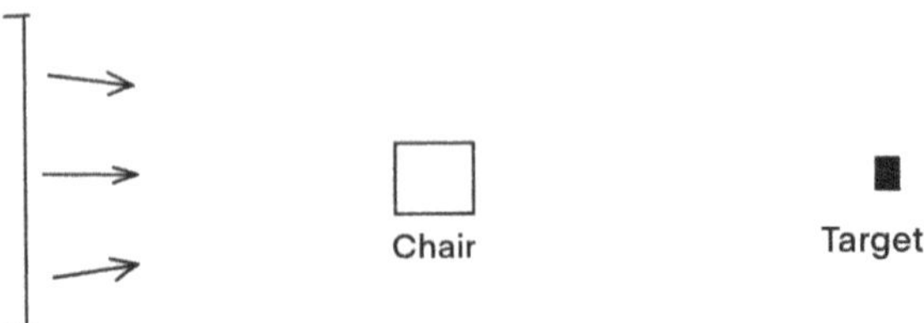

SHOOTING

Feeder – Shooter

One partner is the passer/thrower and the other the goal shooter. The passer throws the ball (feeds it) to the shooter, who on catching the ball shoots at goal. After 10 shots, change positions.

Follow the Leader

With either a shared ball or a ball each, partners take it in turn to lead. The leader does a type of shot the follower must copy:

- → right hand
- → left hand
- → both hands
- → jump shot
- → step and shoot

Around the Clock

Partners take turns to shoot from the 9 o'clock to 3 o'clock positions. What is the best score from these positions?

Ten or Twenty Up

Take turns to shoot from various positions, changing angles and distance. After an equal number of shots from each position, whoever first gets to the target or end number of goals is the winner.

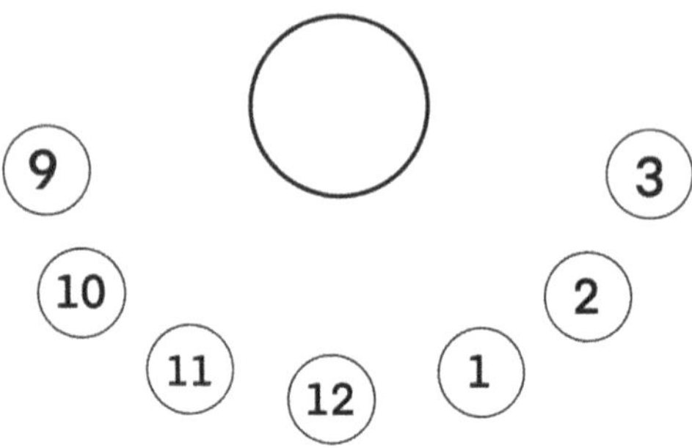

Rebound

One partner shoots and the other catches the rebound no matter if it is a goal or not. They then shoot for goal from the catching spot.

One on One

One partner shoots past a partner's defensive hand and arm. This shooting should vary: over, around, in front, behind.

PIVOT

Follow the Leader

→ One partner does a type of pivot and the other partner has to do the same:
  - left foot
  - right foot
  - jump – land – pivot.

→ This can be done with one partner following the other, or by mirroring, which is doing the same pivot at exactly the same time and speed as each other.
  - The leader chooses the type of movement – then there should be a time of practice.
  - To finish the task, the leader has to give the start signal, and both partners attempt to do the same movement at exactly the same time as each other.

One on One

- → One partner is the defender and the other the attacker.
- → The defender is between the attacker and the target on the wall or the goal.
- → The attacker has to pivot away from defender and pass at the target or shoot for goal.
- → The defender is not allowed to move.
- → Take turns in the two roles.

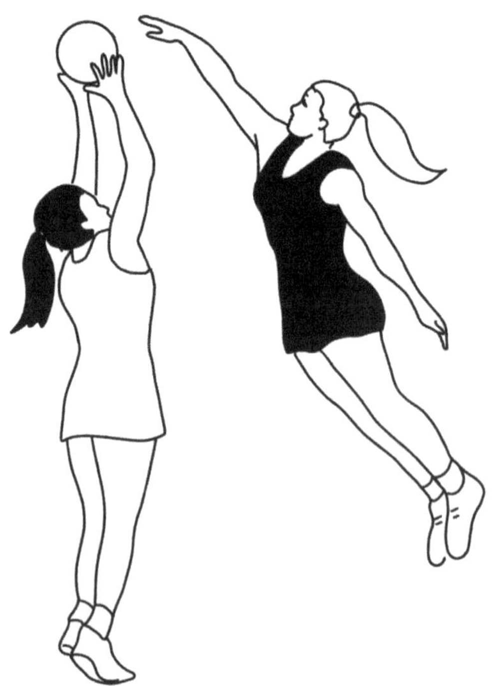

One on one

ATTACK AND DEFEND

Attacking and defending in netball requires the ability to change direction without losing speed or balance.

Follow the Leader

- → Take it in turns to choose agility movements and the other partner follows: run, jump, twist, turn, start, stop.
- → This can be done with one partner following the other or both at the same time (mirroring).

Rhythmic pattern activities

- → Hand clapping, toe tapping, hopping, lunging, swinging arms and legs.
- → These can be done by taking it in turns to choose the activity, one following the other; or mirroring.

Partner matching

- → Rhythmic jumping.
- → Rhythmic jumping with rebounds (very small bounces) between the leaps.
- → Astride jumping.
- → Astride jumping with hand claps.

Knee boxing

- → Facing each other, partners try to tag a knee of each other.
- → Hands can be used to either tag an opponent's knee or to bat away an opponent's hand from their own knee.
- → Grasping a hand is not allowed.
- → First to 10 tags is the winner.

Stepping Stones

- → Mark out a series of circles or lay down a line of hoops.
- → Then hop, jump, leap through the line.
- → This can be made a contest by clean passes (not touching lines) or timing the run throughs

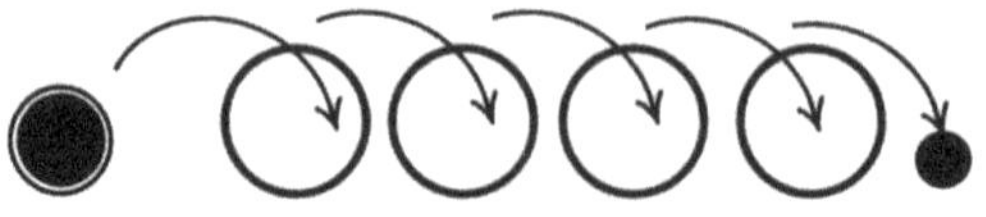

Stepping Stones

Partner skipping games

- → Mirroring
  - ♦ Each partner has their own skipping rope. One partner chooses an activity and the other partner matches (copies/mirrors) it.
  - ♦ All the different types of bounces can be done: plain, rebound, running, crosses, wides, hops, swings, heel-toes.
- → Side by side – one rope shared.
  - ♦ One partner turns the rope with their left hand and the other with their right hand.
  - ♦ All the different bounces can be done.
- → Visiting – a 'call in' game.
  - ♦ One partner skips in their own rope. When the say the 'magic' word, e.g. 'Come in!', the second partner runs in from the front to join them, so now both are skipping facing each other within the same turning rope.
  - ♦ Skipping rhythms – while skipping in unison either mirroring or side by side, the rhymes below are repeated in time to the bouncing beat: For example, Teddy Bear, Teddy Bear, touch the ground.

→ Teddy Bear, Teddy bear, turn around etc.

- Teddy Bear
- Birthday
- Doctor Doctor
- Bluebells.

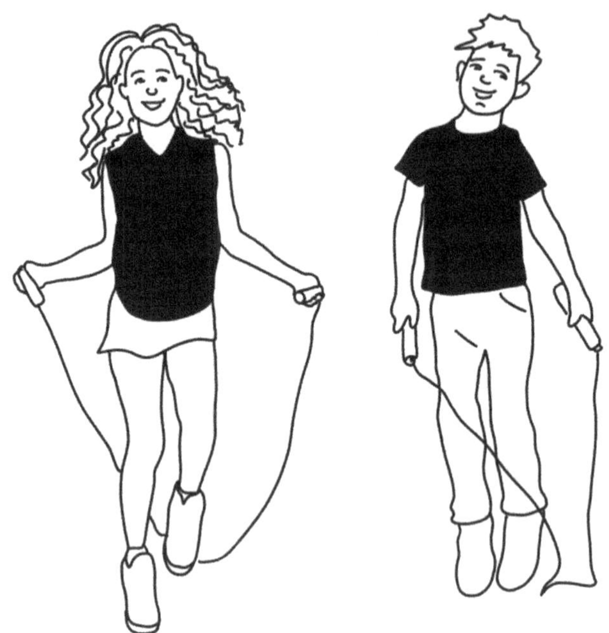

Jump and hop rope

PRACTICE WITH THREE OR MORE

THROW AND CATCH

Set Drills

→ Triangle passing in threes:

- Player A throws to player B, B passes to C, and so on around the triangle. After 10 passes in a clockwise direction, change to 10 passes anticlockwise.

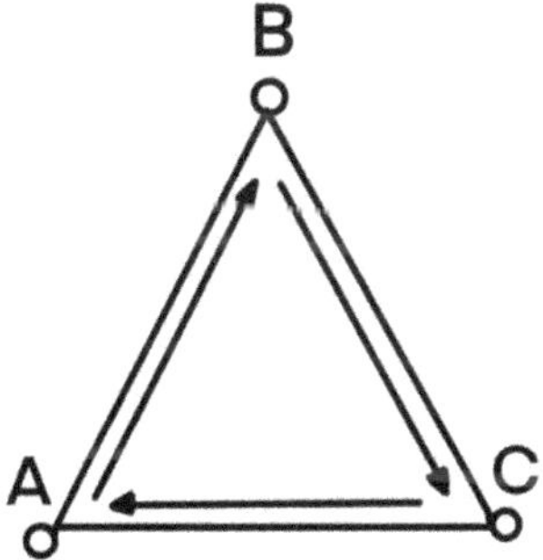

→ Triangle passing in fours:

- Player A passes to player B and immediately follows their throw to take B's place. From a sideline place, D takes A's spot. Player B passes to C and follows their throw. Then C passes to D, and becomes the sideliner.

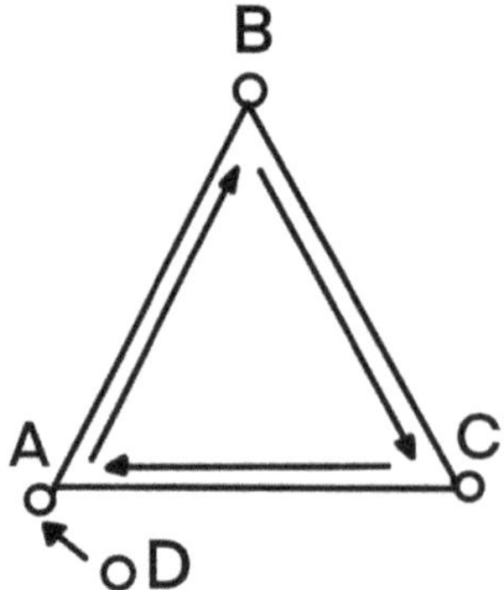

→ Figure of eight

- Starting about 1 metre apart, player A passes to player B, who is running forwards to receive it. Player C is running parallel to B, so then B passes to C. Meanwhile, A has circled around behind B ready to receive the pass from C.
- Players always run behind the player to whom they have passed the ball.
- This is a good practice to move the ball from one end of a court to the other.

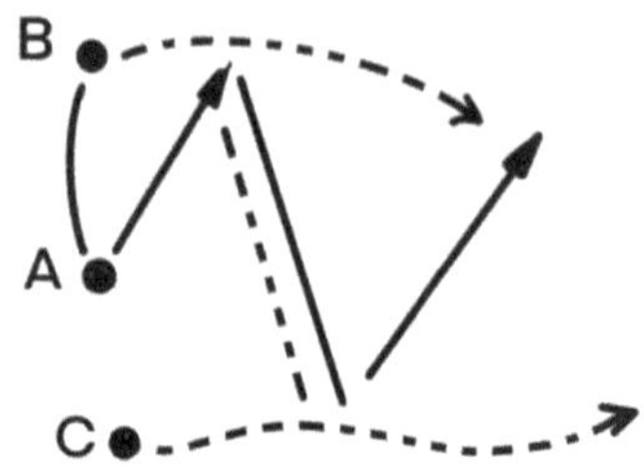

→ Down the line

- Player A passes the ball to player B who is moving sideways.
- Player B pivots after catching the ball and passes to C, who now should be level with B.
- This continues down the line with the ball moving to the right and then left.

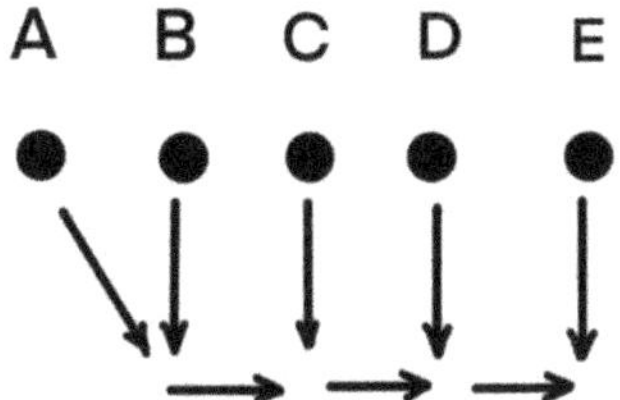

→ Two ways

- Player B runs forwards and receives the ball from player A. Player B then passes it to C and joins onto the end of C's line.
- Player C passes to player A and then A passes to D.
- Player C takes player A's place, and A joins the line where B started.

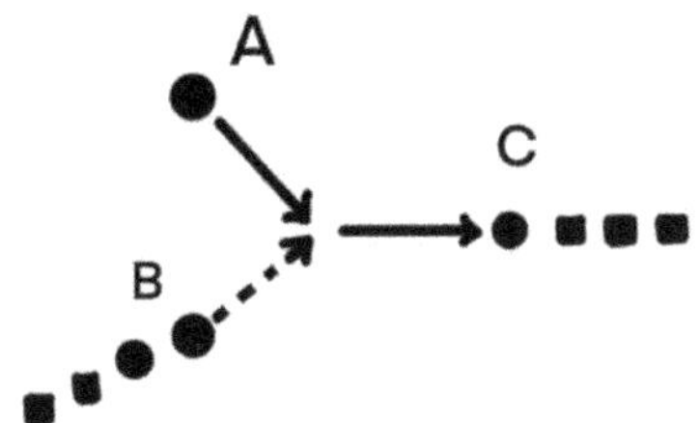

→ Two balls

- Using two balls the passes move up and down the line continuously.
- Player A controls the speed of which the ball moves – this should be as fast as possible without losing control.
- The player 'out the front', player A, has to be throwing one ball as they are receiving the other (the two balls should pass each other in the air).
- This central player should watch the incoming ball and not the one they throw.
- Players B–F in the line are about 1 metre apart, and the central player should be about 2 metres away from this line.

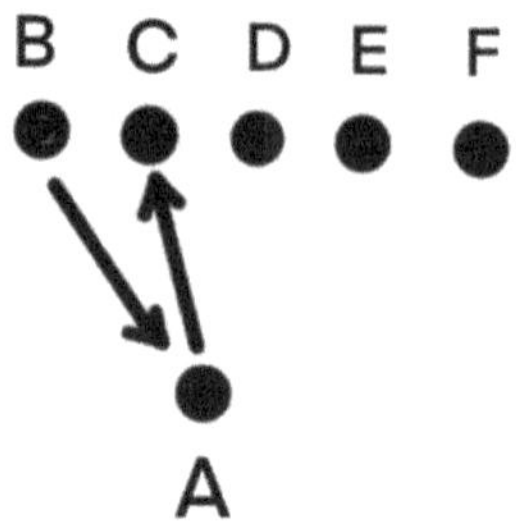

Interception in threes

- Numbers 1 and 3 make as many passes to each other without No. 2 intercepting.

Ten Trips

→ The three players are each 3-4 metres apart.

→ Number 1 throws to No. 3, who passes to No. 2 who in turn passes to No. 1. This circuit is one trip. Circuits continue until there are 10 trips.

→ The three players then rotate positions.

→ This practice can be made more difficult by ruling that if the ball is not caught then that trip cannot be counted in the total.

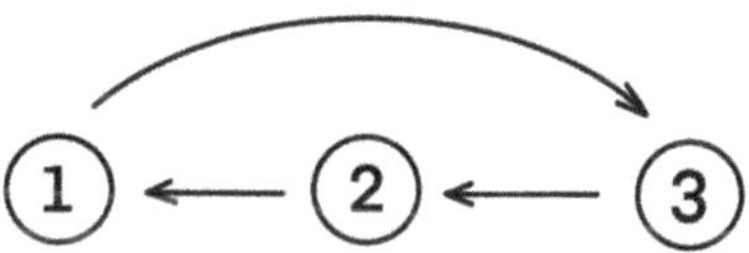

Corner Spry

→ The leader (No. 1) throws the ball and receives it back from players 2–6. The last player in the line (No. 6), on catching the ball runs with it to take up the leader's position.

- At the same time, all players move one place to their right, and the first leader replaces No. 2 in the line.
- This rotation continues until all players have been the leader.

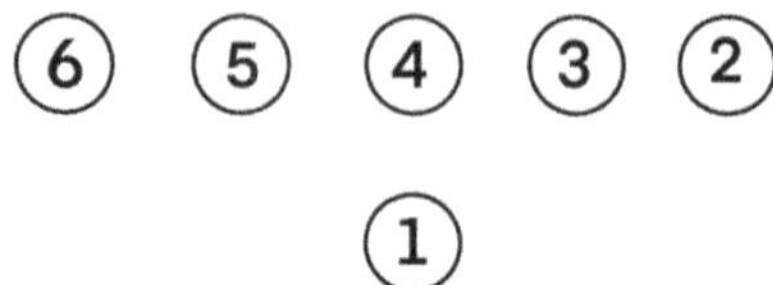

In and Out

- → In a circle formation, the centre player (No. 1) passes the ball and receives it back in order to players 2–6.
- → On receiving the ball, No. 6 runs to the centre and becomes the leader, while the first leader replaces them in the circle.
- → The new centre leader's first pass will be to the player who replaces them in the circle.
- → This process is repeated until all players have had a turn in the centre.

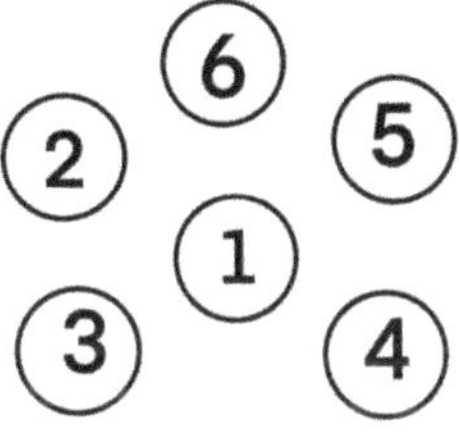

Bob Ball

- → Players in a line, all except the leader facing the same direction (looking at the back of the player in front of them). The leader is facing the opposite way and so is 'face to face' with their teammates.
- → The leader is 2 metres in front of their first teammate.
- → The leader passes the ball and receives it back from the first in line. On returning the ball this player bobs down on their spot.

- The leader then passes over the bobbed team mate to the next in line.
- This process continues until each player has received and returned the ball.
- The game can be extended by having the bobbed players stand up in turn to receive the leaders pass in reverse order.
- It can contain a running part as well.
- The leader passes: 2, 3, 4, 5, 6, then back 6, 5, 4, 3, 2.
- On receiving the ball on its return rotation, No. 2 keeps the ball, runs around the line of players and replaces the leader.
- The initial leader replaces the runner on their spot and the process continues until all players have been to the front to be the leader.

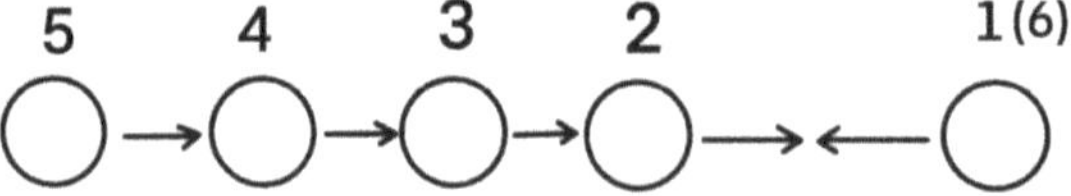

Cross Ball

→ Players are spaced alternately 3 metres apart.

→ Number 1 passes to No. 2, then 2–3, 3–4, 4–5, 5–6, 6–7, 7–8, 8–9, 9–10.

→ Then the passing returns back along the line: 10–9, 9–8, 8–7, etc. The practice ends when the ball is back with No. 1.

→ To increase the difficulty of this practice, the number of times the ball completes the circuit can be increased and the sequence timed.

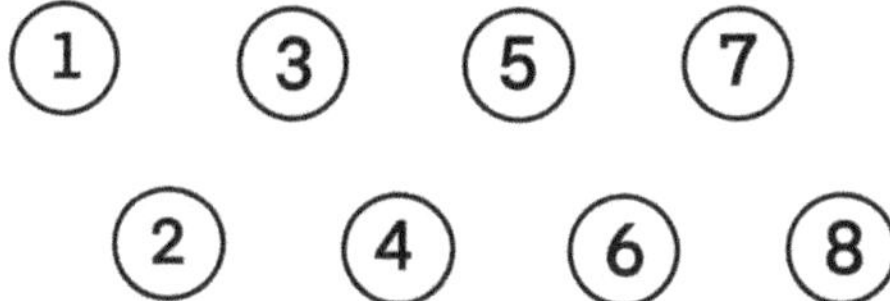

Five in a Row

→ Teams of five players in one-third of a netball court. The team with the ball tries to pass and catch five times without the opposition even touching the ball.

→ The netball rules of stepping, contact, and obstruction apply.

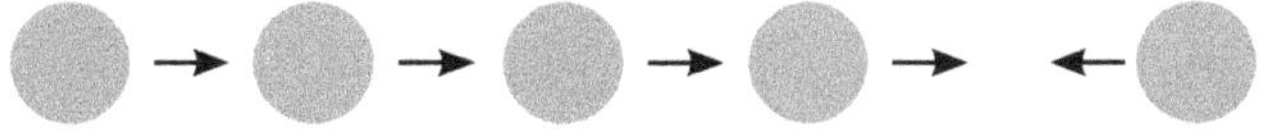

Shooting

Shooting practices for groups are much the same as for pairs.

→ Follow the leader

- Players take it in turn to be leader.
- The leader does a type of shot that all following must copy. This can be one hand, both hands, jump shot, step and shoot.

→ 10 Up

- Players take turns from nominated set positions – changing angles and distance to increase difficulty.
- After an equal number of shots, whoever gets 10 goals first is the winner.

→ School Day Clock

- The first player shoots from the 9 o'clock position, then 10 o'clock, 11, 12, 1, 2, 3.
- Each player follows this procedure.

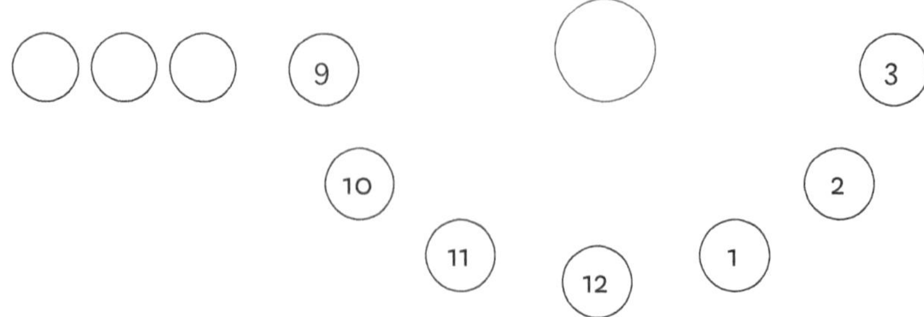

LEAD-UP GAMES

Mat Ball

- → Equal teams of 4–6.
- → Teams take it in turns to start with the ball and start play from a marked centre circle.
- → Using passing and the one-step rule as in netball, teams try to get the ball to their goal shooter who is standing on a mat.
- → This scores one point.
- → The goalie (goal shooter) is not allowed off the mat and no one else is allowed on it.
- → Any loss of possession has the opposition team start from the centre circle again.

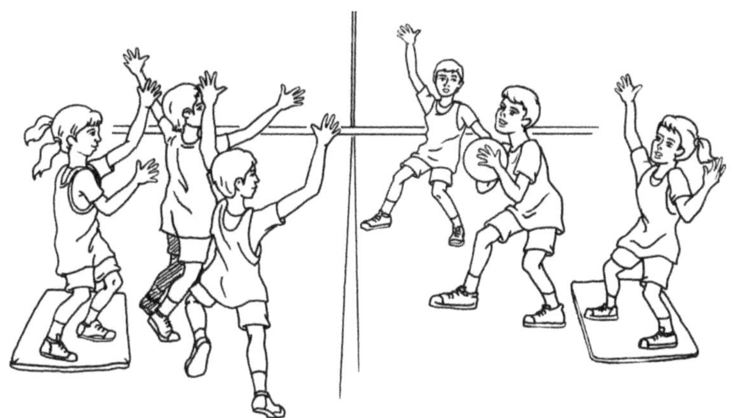

Corner Ball

- → The game is started with a toss-up in the centre circle.
- → Players can then pass the ball but cannot run with it.
- → Players attempt to pass the ball to their team-mates to score a goal.
- → If the ball goes out of bounds, the last touch rule applies (the last team to touch the ball before it goes out loses possession).
- → The other team restarts play with a throw from the sideline.
- → After each goal, play restarts with a centre pass by the non-scoring team.

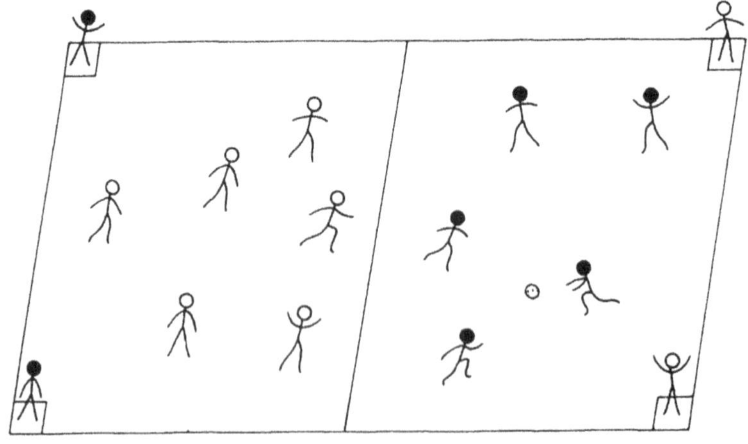

End Ball

- This game needs a playing area of between 12m x 6m to 24 m x 12 m. This is then divided into two end zones and two team zones.
- The two teams of equal numbers each have a goal area where they have three players acting as catchers, and a playing area in which they can move freely without the ball, but not enter the opposition playing area.
- The game is started with a throw-up at the centre circle. The team winning possession of the ball can then pass the ball between themselves with the aim of getting into a position where they can lob the ball over their opponents to be caught by one of their own catchers.
- A player cannot move more than one step when they have possession of the ball.

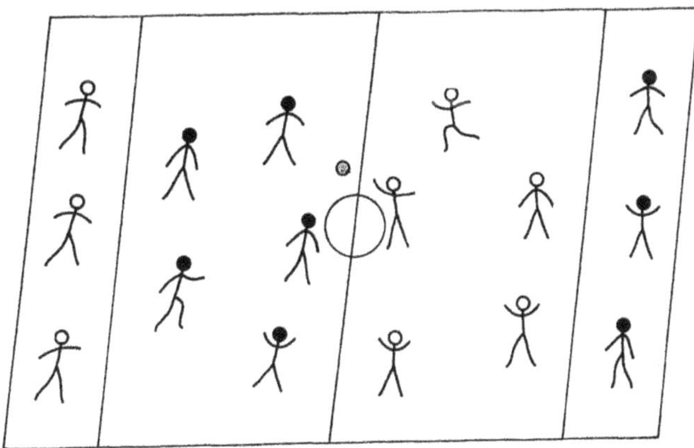

→ If the ball is intercepted, the other team attempts to get the ball to their catchers. If the ball goes out of bounds, the team loses possession.

Invaders

→ For a playing area use two-thirds of a netball court – players are positioned in two divided opposite areas.

→ One player from each team is sent into the opposite area to be an 'invader'.

→ The aim of the game is to get the ball to the invader in this opposite area. When a successful pass has been made to an invader, an additional invader also goes into the opposite area.

→ Scoring starts only when three invaders are in an opponent's area. Points are then scored for each successful pass to an invader.

→ Rules are as for netball.

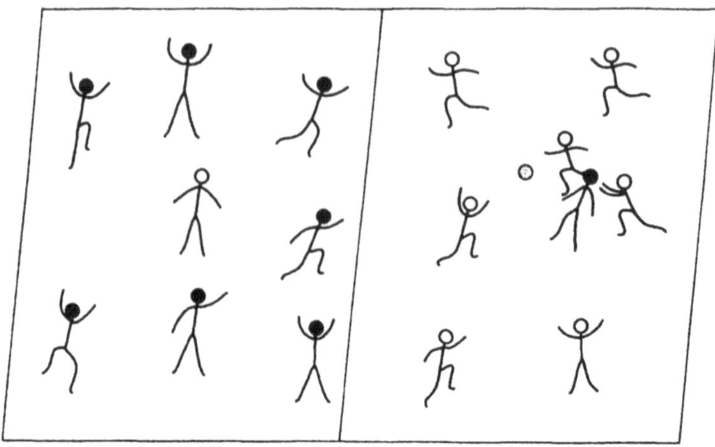

Permit Ball

- → The playing area is the centre third and one forward third of a netball court. (perhaps draw the whole court in diagram below to show only part of the court is used)
- → The game is started with a pass from the permit area.
- → Players then pass the ball until they are able to pass it to the goal shooter, who is then allowed to shoot for a goal.
- → If the ball is intercepted, two of the intercepting team replace the existing permit and goal players and the other team begins a new attack.
- → Stepping and player movement rules are as for netball.

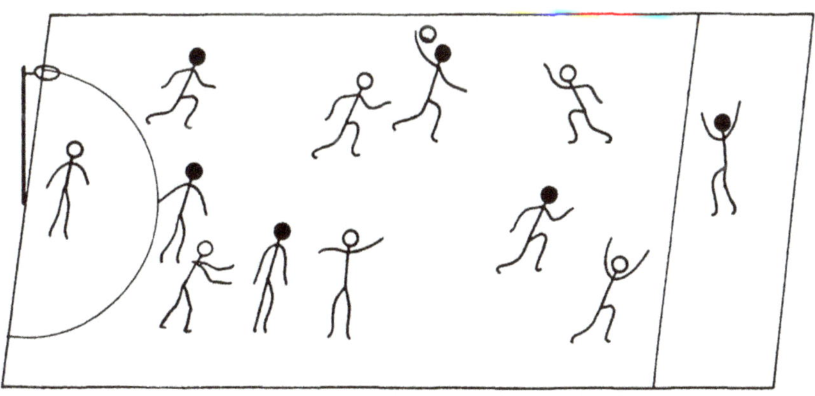

Korfball

- → The game can be played on a netball court, but the playing area is divided into halves instead of thirds.
- → Four players from a team are in one-half of the court and the other four in the other half.
- → One half is a team's defensive half and that contains their goal ring.
- → Players score by throwing a goal in their opposition's half.
- → After two goals, the teams change halves: defenders become attackers and attackers become defenders.
- → Other than when there is a change of halves, attackers cannot go into their defending half, and vice versa.
- → Netball rules apply.

MODIFIED NETBALL

→ Fun Net
- For 5–7-year-olds.
- There are no winners or losers.
- There is no competition.
- Goal posts are 2.4 metres.
- Smaller ball is used (size 4).
- Leaders (parents or teachers) give the children 20–30-minute sessions:
  - warm up and stretches
  - skill practices
  - mini game – 10 minutes.

→ Netta Netball
- For 8–10-year-olds.
- Goal posts are 2.4 metres.
- Smaller ball is used (size 4).
- Game time – four 10-minute quarters.
- Players allowed 6 seconds between catching and throwing.
- Correct footwork encouraged.

- Defenders must be 1.2 metres from the player with the ball.
- No defence is allowed on a shot for goal.

→ High Five Netball

- For 9–11-year-olds.
- Only five positions: goal shooter, goal attack, centre, goal defence, goalkeeper.
- Players allowed 4 seconds between catching and throwing.
- Correct footwork is enforced.
- No outstretched arms permitted in defence.
- Permitted zones for player positions:
    - GS – attacking and centre thirds
    - GA – attacking and centre thirds
    - C – all areas except the two goal circles
    - GD – centre and defensive thirds
    - GK – centre and defensive thirds.

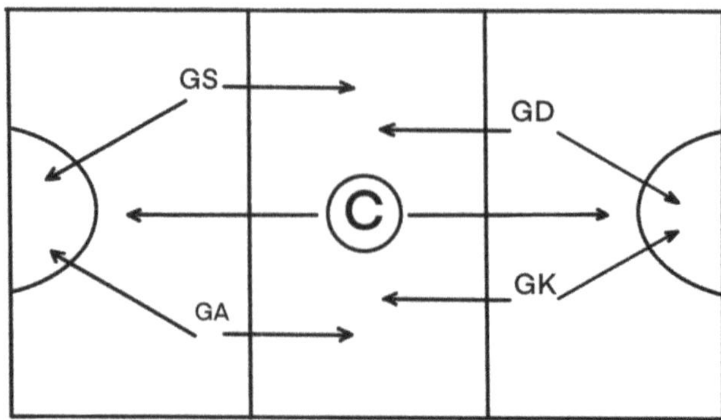

Player zones

SENIOR NETBALL

Basic Rules

- → Seven players per team.
- → Players restricted to zones:
  - GS – all front thirds
  - GA – all front and centre thirds
  - WA – front, and centre thirds but not the goal circle
  - C – front, centre and back thirds but no goal circles
  - WD – back and centre thirds but not the goal circle
  - GD – all back and centre thirds
  - GK – all back third
- → Only the goal shooter and the goal attack are permitted to shoot for goal.
- → Goals can only be scored from within the goal circle.
- → A match consists of four 15-minute quarters.
- → The umpire is in total control of the match.
- → Players cannot hold the ball for longer than 3 seconds.
- → Each quarter is started and play after a goal is restarted by a centre pass.

- → After a ball goes out of play over the sidelines, play is restarted by a throw-in by the team other than the one that last touched the ball.
- → After a disputed ball, play is restarted with a toss-up between the two players concerned.
- → A defender's feet must be at least 0.9 metres from the attacker with the ball. Being closer leads to an obstruction penalty of a free pass.
- → Stepping – a player cannot take more than one step after gaining possession of the ball.
- → A player is off-side if they enter a playing area other than their allocated zone.

Players' roles:

- → Goal shooter
  - Restricted to the attacking third of the court and has the major responsibility for scoring goals.
  - Usually a tall player.
- → Goal attack
  - Provides the link from the middle third into the attacking third.
  - Is the second player that can shoot for goal.
  - This player needs speed and mobility.

- → Wing attack
  - the link player between the middle and attacking third, but is not allowed in the goal circle.
  - A player who can get free easily to receive a pass.
- → Centre
  - Covers all three thirds but is not allowed into the goal circles.
  - This player is involved with most play and has therefore got to have stamina.
  - Their aim is to control the pace of their attacking play and delay that of the opposing team.
- → Wing defence
  - Probably has the most difficult role. Defends the opposition wing attack player.
  - Needs speed and judgement, and should be an expert passer of the ball themselves.
- → Goal defence
  - Covers the defensive and middle thirds.
  - Must be able to defend and attack.
- → Goalkeeper
  - The main defender in the defensive third and goal circle.
  - Usually tall and can jump high.

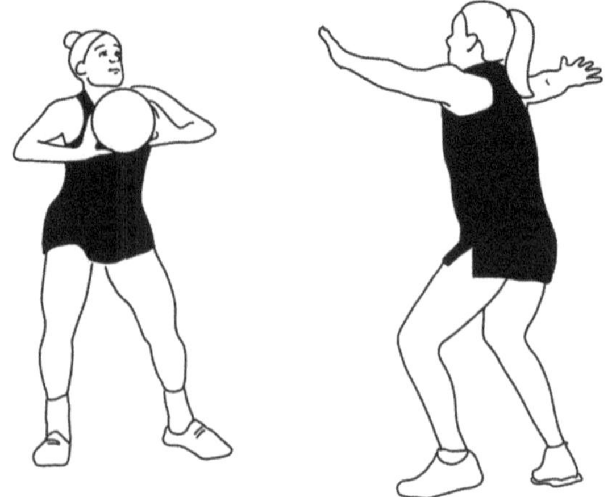

Wing attack versus wing defence

WARM UP AND WARM DOWN

→ **Jogging**

- on the spot
- slow runs forwards
- slow runs backwards

→ **Neck and shoulders**

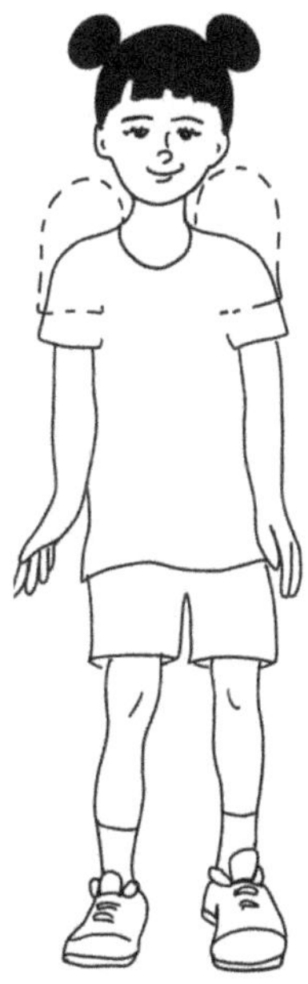

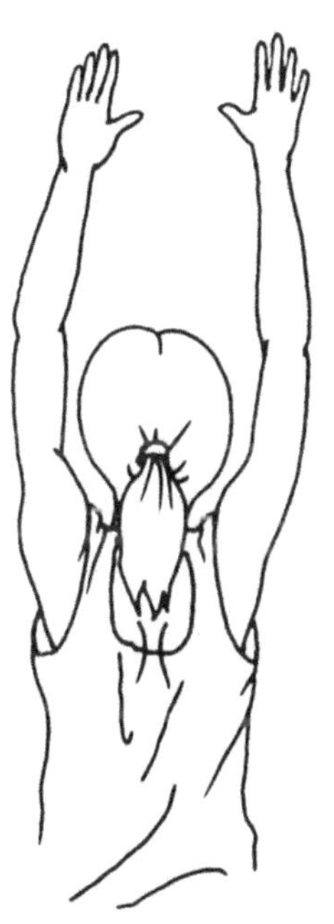

- Stand with feet shoulder width apart, shrug shoulders near to ears – left, right, both.

- With arms raised, move shoulder blades closer together.

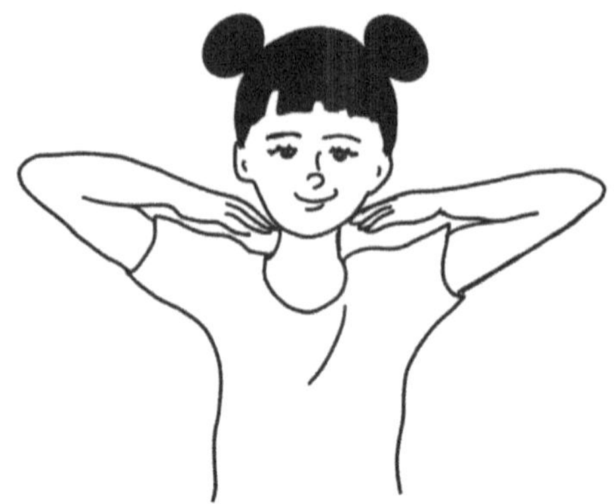

- With fingers touching the neck, elbows pressed back – rotate the elbows forwards and then backwards – left, right, both.

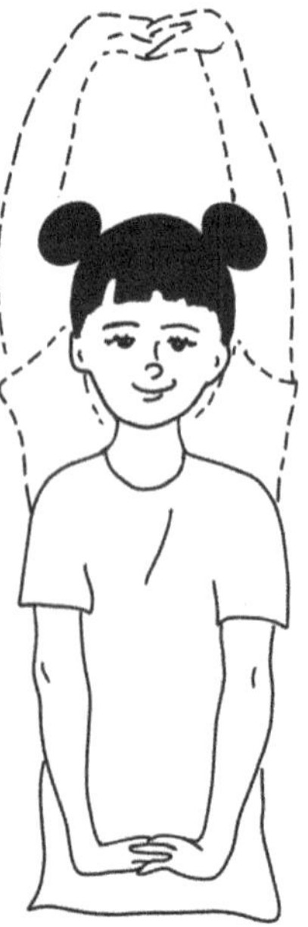

- With fingers interlaced, palms down, back straight – press hands downwards for the count of four; then with hands above head and palms up, press upwards for the count of four.

→ **Trunk and arms**

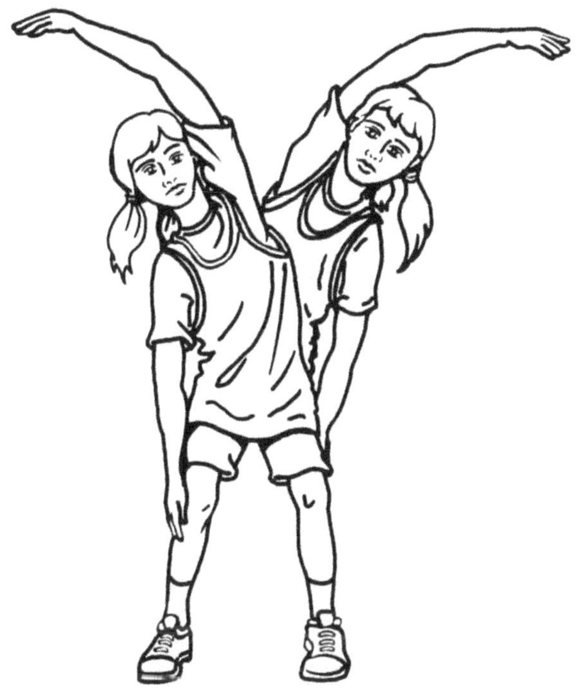

- Side stretching – feet shoulder width apart, one arm held high with palm inwards; opposite arm held down with palm along thigh: bend the trunk slowly sidewards to slide palm down the leg, then return to vertical. Repeat to opposite side with a change of arms – left, right alternate.

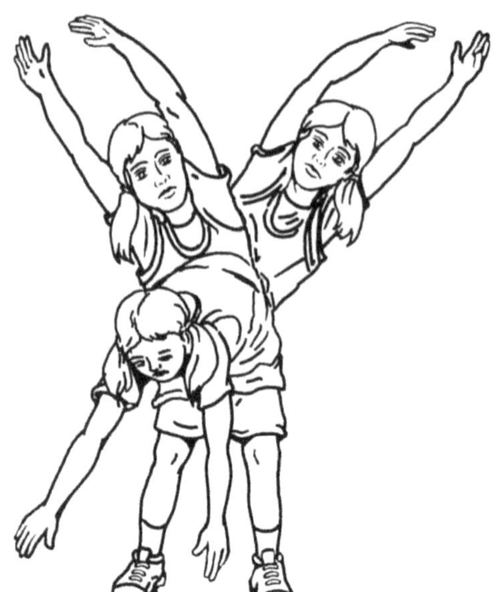

- Trunk circling – with arms above head, circle arms to the right in slow sweeping movements with hands passing low, at least at knee level.
- Repeat to the left, then alternate.

- Arm circles – with arms straight, and standing erect, make arm circles – right arm, left arm, both arms alternate. First done swinging forwards and then backwards.

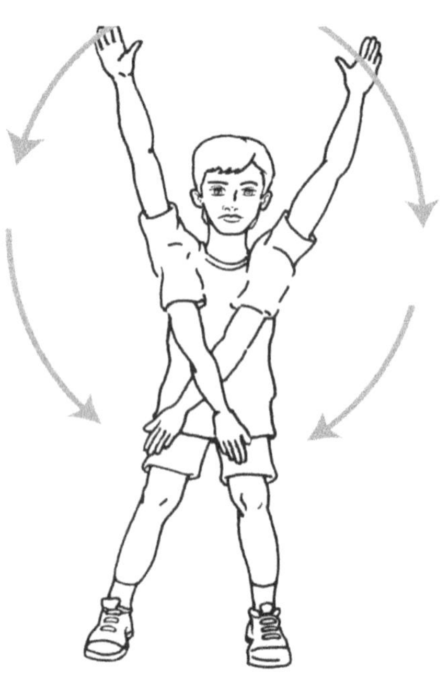

→ Legs and back

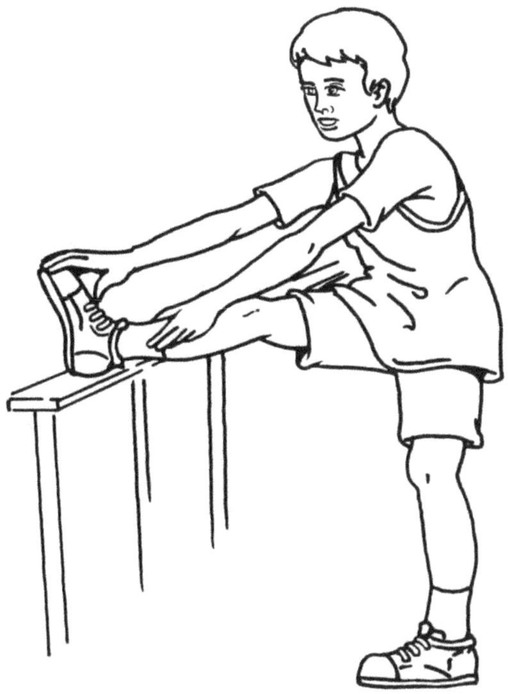

- Hamstring stretch – one leg with heel placed on support between knee and groin high, toe pointing up. Lean the body gently forwards until a slight stretch can be felt in the hamstring. This position is held for 5–10 seconds, then the body returns to the start position. This is repeated 5–10 times, and then same process for the other leg.

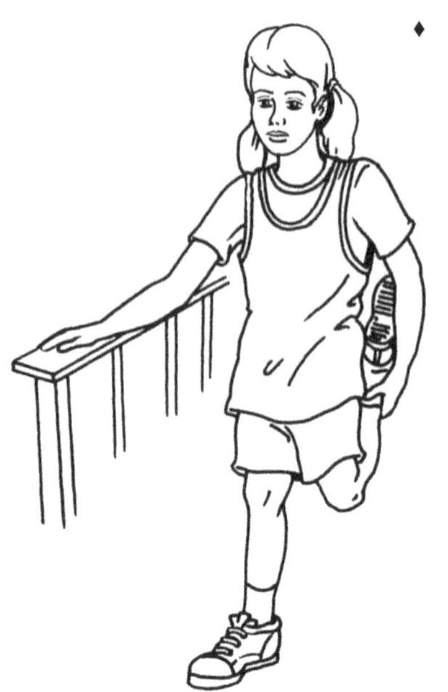

- Quadriceps stretch – one hand holding a support, and standing on one leg (the same side as the support arm). The opposite foot is held near the ankle and then the foot is gently pulled towards the buttock until a slight stretch is felt. This position is held for 5–10 seconds, then returns to the starting position and then the same process for the other leg.

- Calf stretch – facing a wall and with palms against it. Put one foot in front of the other, front knee slightly bent and back knee straight but with the heel on the ground. The front knee is gently bent further until a slight stretch can be felt in the calf of the back leg. Hold for 5–10 seconds with 5–10 repetitions, then repeat using the other leg.

www.ingramcontent.com/pod-product-compliance
Ingram Content Group Australia Pty Ltd
76 Discovery Rd, Dandenong South VIC 3175, AU
AUHW020731051125
418993AU00001B/1

9 781922 872180